My Air Fryer Breakfast

Tasty and Affordable Air Fryer Recipes to Start Your Day with the Right Foot

Eva Sheppard

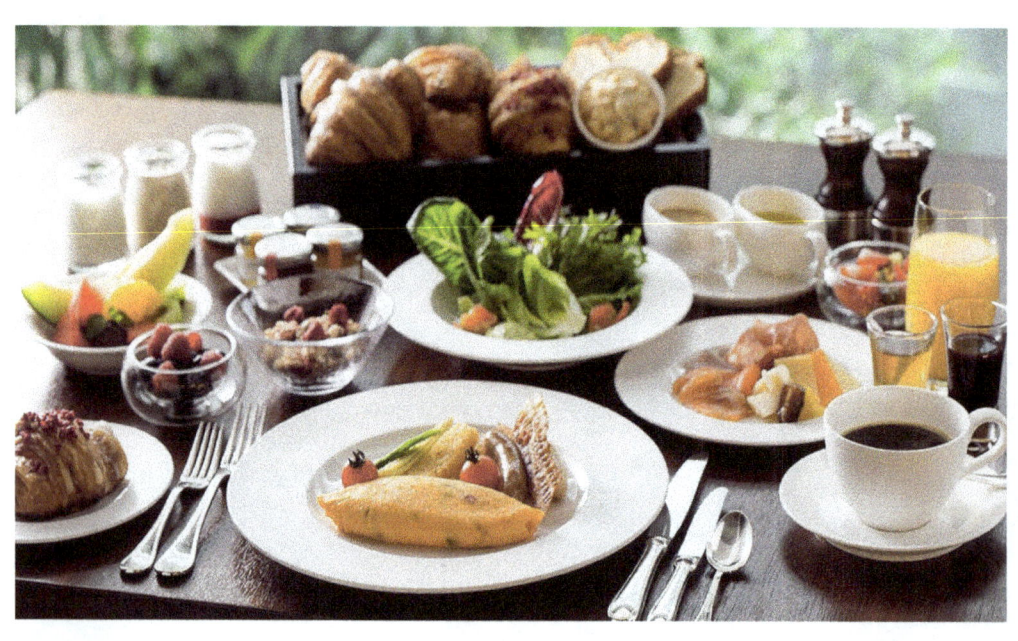

© **Copyright 2021 - All rights reserved.**

The content contained within this book may not be reproduced, duplicated or transmitted without direct written permission from the author or the publisher.

Under no circumstances will any blame or legal responsibility be held against the publisher, or author, for any damages, reparation, or monetary loss due to the information contained within this book. Either directly or indirectly.

Legal Notice:

This book is copyright protected. This book is only for personal use. You cannot amend, distribute, sell, use, quote or paraphrase any part, or the content within this book, without the consent of the author or publisher.

Disclaimer Notice:

Please note the information contained within this document is for educational and entertainment purposes only. All effort has been executed to present accurate, up to date, and reliable, complete information. No warranties of any kind are declared or implied. Readers acknowledge that the author is not engaging in the rendering of legal, financial, medical or professional advice. The content within this book has been derived from various sources. Please consult a licensed professional before attempting any techniques outlined in this book.

By reading this document, the reader agrees that under no circumstances is the author responsible for any losses, direct or indirect, which are incurred as a result of the use of information contained within this document, including, but not limited to, — errors, omissions, or inaccuracies.

TABLE OF CONTENT

Blackberries and Cornflakes *8*
Fried Mushroom *9*
Pancakes *12*
Creamy Mushroom Pie *14*
Pear Oatmeal *17*
Ham and Cheese Patties *19*
Peppers and Lettuce Salad *20*
Cod Tortilla *22*
Artichoke Omelet *24*
Carrot Oatmeal *25*
Chicken Burrito *26*
Potato Frittata *29*
Herbed Omelet *31*
Cheese Toast *32*
Carrots and Cauliflower Mix *33*
Vanilla Oatmeal *35*
Fish Tacos Breakfast *36*
Tuna Sandwiches *39*
Tofu and Bell Peppers *41*
Cheering Chicken Sandwiches *42*
Chicken Pie Recipe *44*
Dill and Scallops *46*

Cheesy Ravioli and Marinara Sauce 47

Cheese and Macaroni 50

Zucchini and Tuna Tortillas 53

Beef Meatballs 55

Easy Egg Muffins 57

Breakfast Potatoes 58

Breakfast Ham Dish 61

Banana Oatmeal Casserole 64

Tasty Polenta Bites 66

Eggs and Tomatoes 67

Fried Sandwich 70

Breakfast Casserole 71

Cheese Fried Bake 73

Delightful Eggs Casserole 75

Morning Egg Bowls 77

Thyme Potato Breakfast Mix 80

Chicken and Spinach Breakfast Casserole 82

Sausage Bake 84

Breakfast Chicken Burrito 86

Fruity Breakfast Casserole 88

Smoked Bacon and Bread Mix 90

Cheesy Hash Brown Mix 92

Roasted Peppers Frittata 94

Blackberries and Cornflakes Mix 96

.... 99

Simple Scrambled Eggs..100
Creamy Mushroom Pie 101
Carrots and Cauliflower Breakfast Mix 103
Delicious Doughnuts...105

Blackberries and Cornflakes

Preparation Time: 15 minutes

Servings: 4

Ingredients:
- 3 cups milk
- 1/4 cup blackberries
- 2 eggs; whisked
- 1 tbsp. sugar
- 1/4 tsp. nutmeg; ground
- 4 tbsp. cream cheese; whipped
- 1½ cups corn flakes

Directions:
1. In a bowl, mix all ingredients and stir well.
2. Heat up your air fryer at 350°F, add the corn flakes mixture, spread and cook for 10 minutes. Divide between plates, serve and enjoy

Fried Mushroom

Preparation Time: 25 minutes

Servings: 4

Ingredients:

- 7 oz. spinach; torn
- 8 cherry tomatoes; halved
- 4 slices bacon; chopped.
- 4 eggs
- 8 white mushrooms; sliced
- 1 garlic clove; minced
- A drizzle of olive oil
- Salt and black pepper to taste

Directions:

1. In a pan greased with oil and that fits your air fryer, mix all ingredients except for the spinach; stir.

2. Put the pan in your air fryer and cook at 400°F for 15 minutes. Add the spinach, toss

and cook for 5 minutes more. Divide between plates and serve

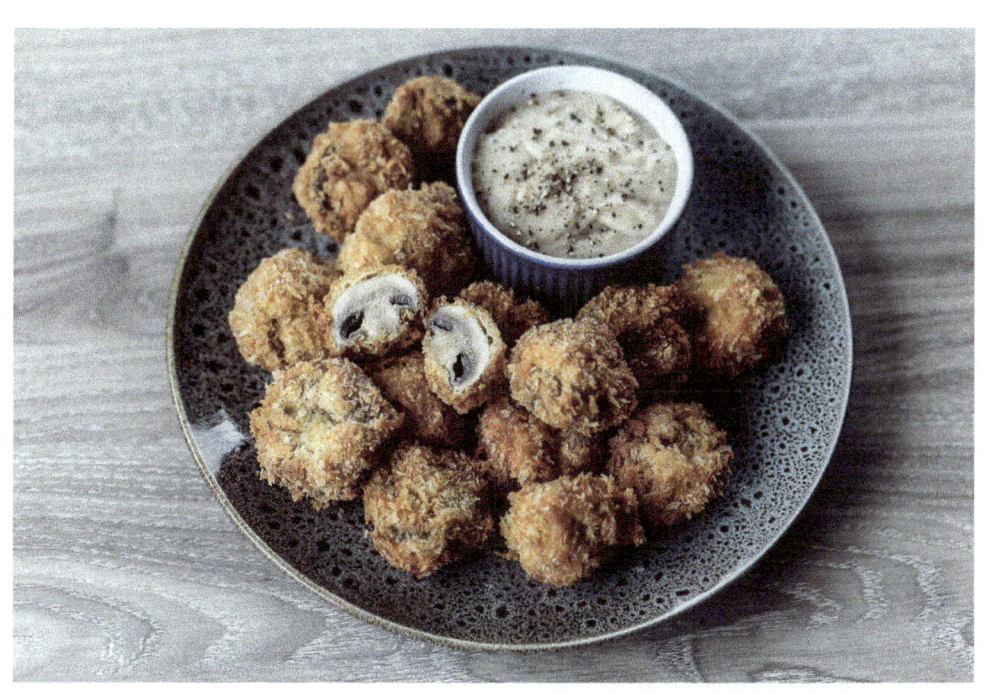

Pancakes

Preparation Time: 30 minutes

Servings: 4

Ingredients:

- 1¾ cups white flour
- 1 cup apple; peeled, cored and chopped.
- 1¼ cups milk
- 1 egg; whisked
- 2 tbsp. sugar
- 2 tsp. baking powder
- 1/4 tsp. vanilla extract
- 2 tsp. cinnamon powder
- Cooking spray

Directions:

1. In a bowl, mix all ingredients -except cooking sprayand stir until you obtain a smooth batter

2. Grease your air fryer's pan with the cooking spray and pour in 1/4 of the batter; spread it into the pan.
3. Cover and cook at 360°F for 5 minutes, flipping it halfway
4. Repeat steps 2 and 3 with 1/4 of the batter 3 more times and then serve the pancakes right away.

Creamy Mushroom Pie

Preparation Time: 20 minutes

Servings: 4

Ingredients:

- 6 white mushrooms; chopped.
- 3 eggs
- 1 red onion; chopped.
- 9-inch pie dough
- 1/4 cup cheddar cheese; grated
- 1/2 cup heavy cream
- 2 tbsp. bacon; cooked and crumbled
- 1 tbsp. olive oil
- 1/2 tsp. thyme; dried
- Salt and black pepper to taste

Directions:

1. Roll the dough on a working surface, then press it on the bottom of a pie pan that fits your air fryer and grease with the oil

2. In a bowl, mix all other ingredients except the cheese, stir well and pour mixture into the pie pan

3. Sprinkle the cheese on top, put the pan in the air fryer and cook at 400°F for 10 minutes. Slice and serve.

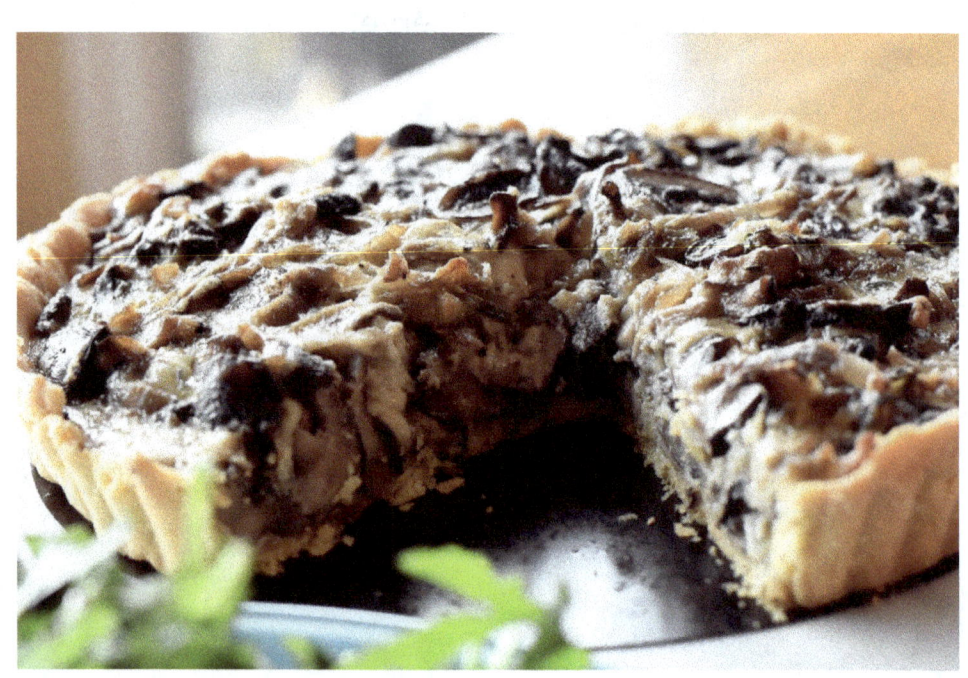

Pear Oatmeal

Preparation Time: 17 minutes

Servings: 4

Ingredients:

- 1 cup milk
- 1/4 cups brown sugar
- 1/2 cup walnuts; chopped.
- 2 cups pear; peeled and chopped.
- 1 cup old fashioned oats
- 1/2 tsp. cinnamon powder
- 1 tbsp. butter; softened

Directions:

1. In a heat-proof bowl that fits your air fryer, mix all ingredients and stir well. Place in your fryer and cook at 360°F for 12 minutes. Divide into bowls and serve

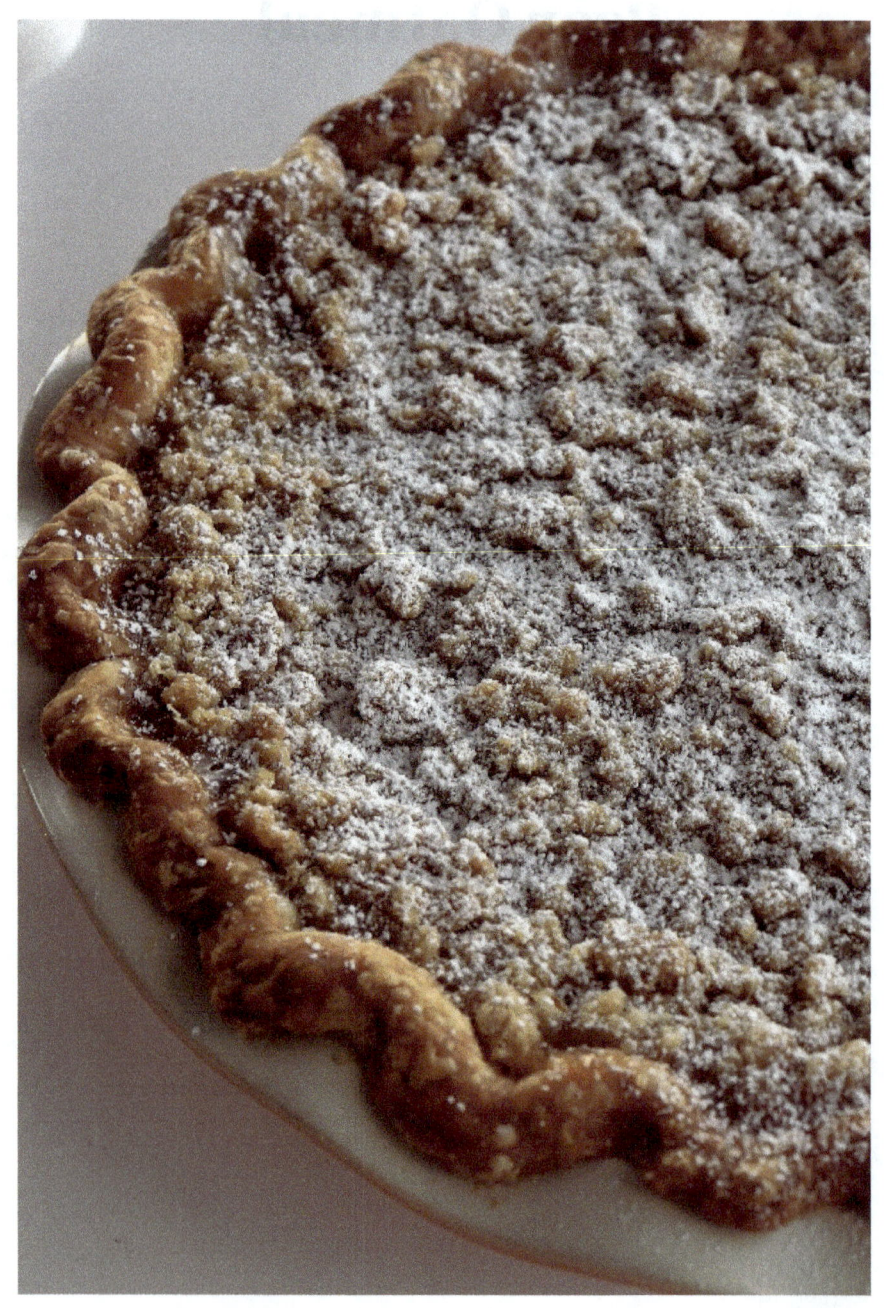

Ham and Cheese Patties

Preparation Time: 20 minutes

Servings: 4

Ingredients:

- 8 ham slices; chopped.
- 4 handfuls mozzarella cheese; grated
- 1 puff pastry sheet
- 4 tsp. mustard

Directions:

2. Roll out puff pastry on a working surface and cut it in 12 squares. Divide cheese, ham and mustard on half of them, top with the other halves and seal the edges
3. Place all the patties in your air fryer's basket and cook at 370°F for 10 minutes. Divide the patties between plates and serve

Peppers and Lettuce Salad

Preparation Time: 15 minutes

Servings: 4

Ingredients:

- 2 oz. rocket leaves
- 4 red bell peppers
- 1 lettuce head; torn
- 2 tbsp. olive oil
- 1 tbsp. lime juice
- 3 tbsp. heavy cream
- Salt and black pepper to taste

Directions:

1. Place the bell peppers in your air fryer's basket and cook at 400°F for 10 minutes
2. Remove the peppers, peel, cut them into strips and put them in a bowl. Add all remaining ingredients, toss and serve

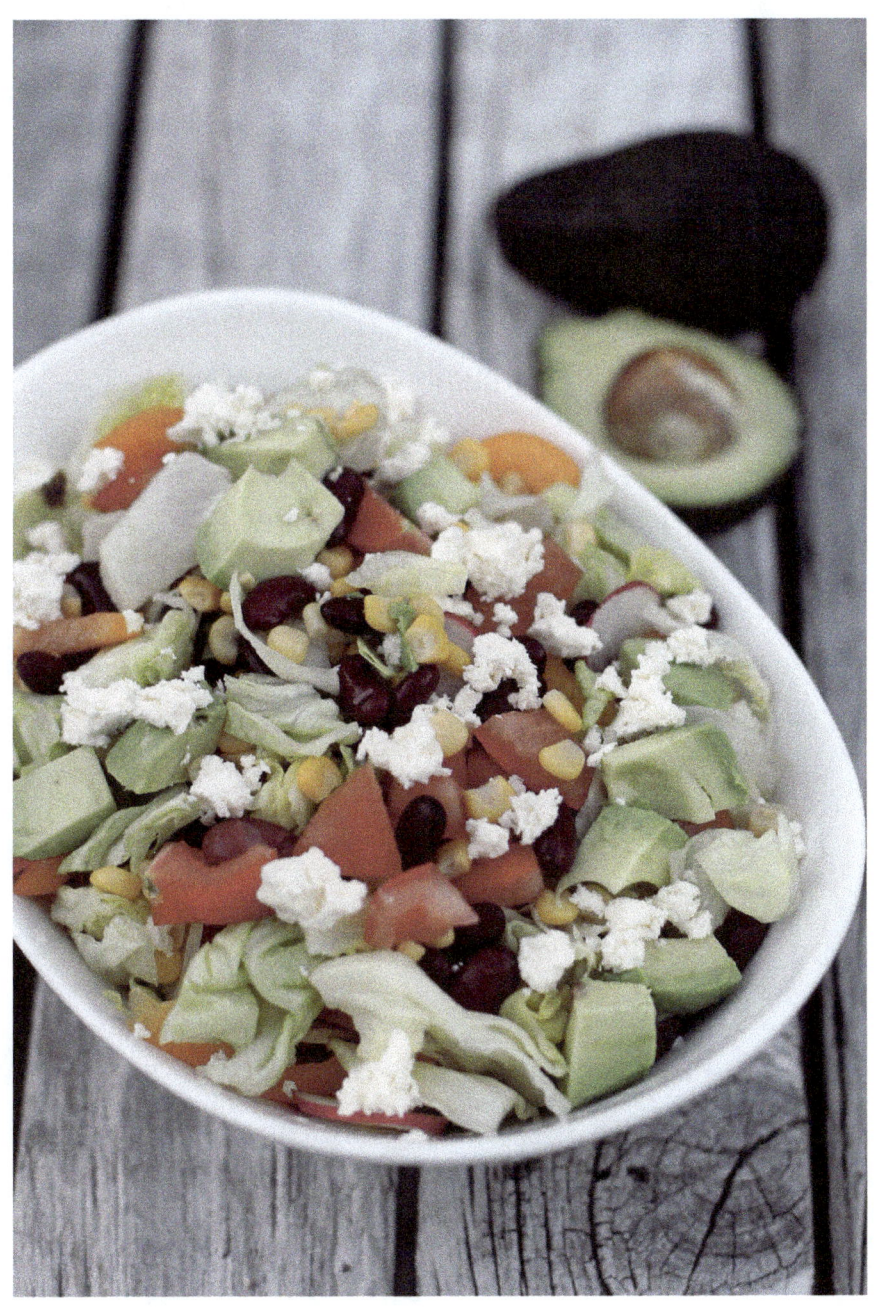

Cod Tortilla

Preparation Time: 27 minutes

Servings: 4

Ingredients:

- 4 cod fillets; skinless and boneless
- 4 tortillas
- 1 green bell pepper; chopped.
- 1 red onion; chopped.
- A drizzle of olive oil
- 1 cup corn
- 1/2 cup salsa
- 4 tbsp. parmesan cheese; grated
- A handful of baby spinach

Directions:

1. Put the fish fillets in your air fryer's basket, cook at 350°F for 6 minutes and transfer to a plate.

2. Heat up a pan with the oil over medium heat, add the bell peppers, onions and corn and stir

3. Sauté for 5 minutes and take off the heat. Arrange all the tortillas on a working surface and divide the cod, salsa, sautéed veggies, spinach and parmesan evenly between the 4 tortillas; then wrap / roll them

4. Place the tortillas in your air fryer's basket and cook at 350°F for 6 minutes. Divide between plates, serve.

Artichoke Omelet

Preparation Time: 20 minutes

Servings:

Ingredients:

- 3 artichoke hearts; canned, drained and chopped.
- 6 eggs; whisked
- 2 tbsp. avocado oil
- 1/2 tsp. oregano; dried
- Salt and black pepper to taste

Directions:

1. In a bowl, mix all ingredients except the oil; stir well. Add the oil to your air fryer's pan and heat it up at 320°F.

2. Add the egg mixture, cook for 15 minutes, divide between plates and serve

Carrot Oatmeal

Preparation Time: 20 minutes

Servings: 4

Ingredients:

- 1/2 cup steel cut oats
- 2 cups almond milk
- 1 cup carrots; shredded
- 2 tsp. sugar
- 1 tsp. cardamom; ground
- Cooking spray

Directions:

1. Spray your air fryer with cooking spray, add all ingredients, toss and cover. Cook at 365°F for 15 minutes. Divide into bowls and serve

Chicken Burrito

Preparation Time: 15 minutes

Servings: 2

Ingredients:

- 4 chicken breast slices; cooked and shredded
- 2 tortillas
- 1 avocado; peeled, pitted and sliced
- 1 green bell pepper; sliced
- 2 eggs; whisked
- 2 tbsp. mild salsa
- 2 tbsp. cheddar cheese; grated
- Salt and black pepper to taste

Directions:

2. In a bowl, whisk the eggs with the salt and pepper and pour them into a pan that fits your air fryer. Put the pan in the air fryer's basket, cook for 5 minutes at 400°F and transfer the mix to a plate

3. Place the tortillas on a working surface and between them divide the eggs, chicken, bell peppers, avocado and the cheese; roll the burritos

4. Line your air fryer with tin foil, add the burritos and cook them at 300°F for 3-4 minutes. Serve for breakfast-or lunch, or dinner!

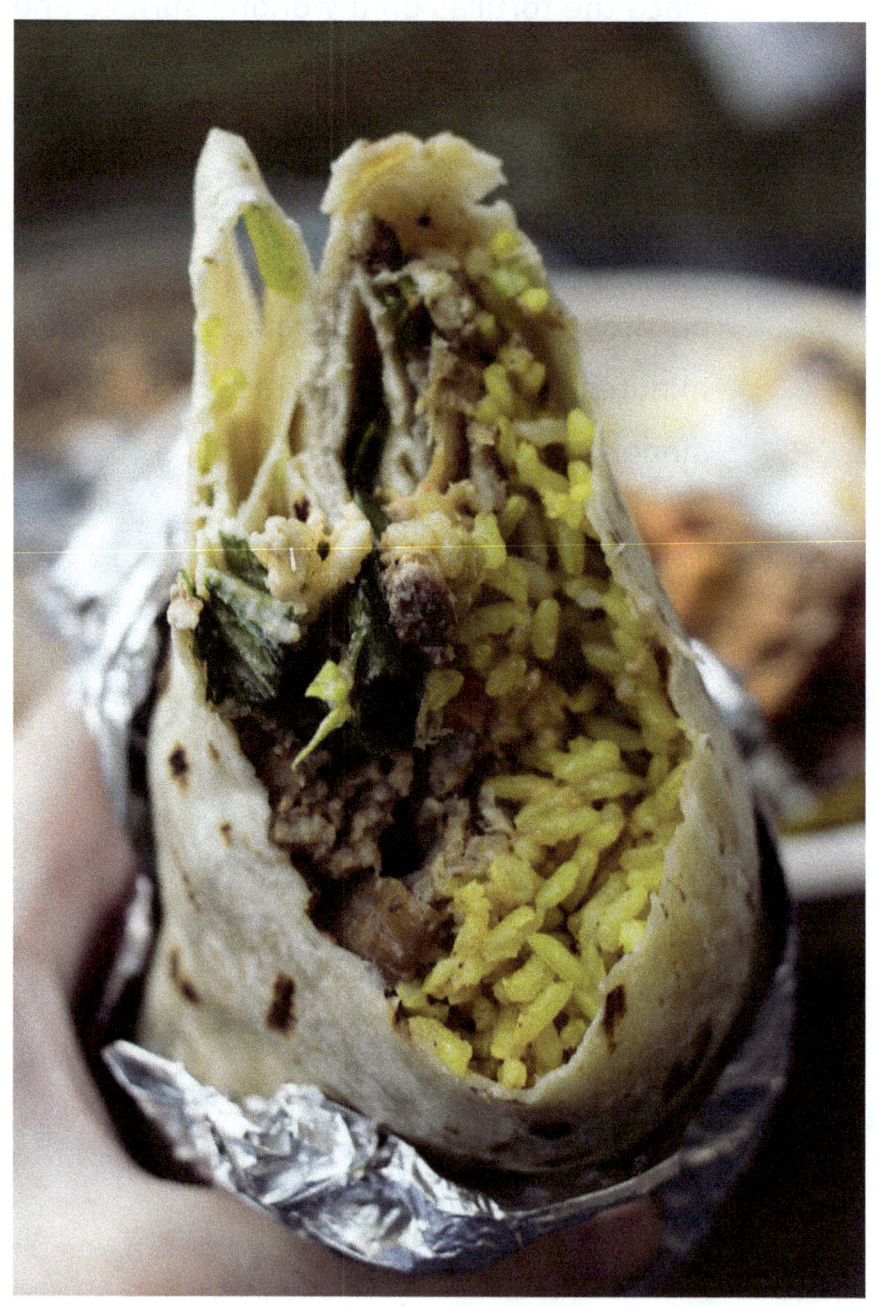

Potato Frittata

Preparation Time: 25 minutes

Servings: 6

Ingredients:

- 1 lb. small potatoes; chopped.
- 1 oz. parmesan cheese; grated
- 1/2 cup heavy cream
- 2 red onions; chopped.
- 8 eggs; whisked
- 1 tbsp. olive oil
- Salt and black pepper to taste

Directions:

1. In a bowl, mix all ingredients except the potatoes and oil; stir well.

2. Heat up your air fryer's pan with the oil at 320°F. Add the potatoes, stir and cook for 5 minutes

3. Add the egg mixture, spread and cook for 15 minutes more. Divide the frittata between plates and serve

Herbed Omelet

Preparation Time: 20 minutes

Servings: 4

Ingredients:

- 6 eggs; whisked
- 2 tbsp. parmesan cheese; grated
- 4 tbsp. heavy cream
- 1 tbsp. parsley; chopped.
- 1 tbsp. tarragon; chopped.
- 2 tbsp. chives; chopped.
- Salt and black pepper to taste

Directions:

1. In a bowl, mix all ingredients except for the parmesan and whisk well. Pour this into a pan that fits your air fryer, place it in preheated fryer and cook at 350°F for 15 minutes

2. Divide the omelet between plates and serve with the parmesan sprinkled on top

Cheese Toast

Preparation Time: 13 minutes

Servings: 2

Ingredients:

- 4 bread slices
- 4 cheddar cheese slices
- 4 tsp. butter; softened

Directions:

1. Spread the butter on each slice of bread. Place 2 cheese slices each on 2 bread slices, then top with the other 2 bread slices; cut each in half

2. Arrange the sandwiches in your air fryer's basket and cook at 370°F for 8 minutes. Serve hot and enjoy!

Carrots and Cauliflower Mix

Preparation Time: 30 minutes

Servings: 4

Ingredients:

- 1 cauliflower head; stems removed, florets separated and steamed
- 2 oz. milk
- 2 oz. cheddar cheese; grated
- 3 carrots; chopped and steamed
- 3 eggs
- 2 tsp. cilantro; chopped.
- Salt and black pepper to taste

Directions:

1. In a bowl, mix the eggs with the milk, parsley, salt and pepper; whisk. Put the cauliflower and the carrots in your air fryer, add the egg mixture and spread. Then sprinkle the cheese on top

2. Cook at 350°F for 20 minutes, divide between plates and serve

Vanilla Oatmeal

Preparation Time: 22 minutes

Servings: 4

Ingredients:

- 1 cup steel cut oats
- 1 cup milk
- 2½ cups water
- 2 tsp. vanilla extract
- 2 tbsp. brown sugar

Directions:

1. In a pan that fits your air fryer, mix all ingredients and stir well. Place the pan in your air fryer and cook at 360°F for 17 minutes. Divide into bowls and serve

Fish Tacos Breakfast

Preparation Time: 23 Minutes

Servings: 4

Ingredients:

- 4 big tortillas
- 1 yellow onion; chopped
- 1 cup corn
- 1 red bell pepper; chopped
- 1/2 cup salsa
- 4 white fish fillets; skinless and boneless
- A handful mixed romaine lettuce; spinach and radicchio
- 4 tbsp. parmesan; grated

Directions:

1. Put fish fillets in your air fryer and cook at 350°F, for 6 minutes

2. Meanwhile; heat up a pan over medium high heat, add bell pepper, onion and corn; stir and cook for 1 - 2 minutes

3. Arrange tortillas on a working surface, divide fish fillets, spread salsa over them; divide mixed veggies and mixed greens and spread parmesan on each at the end.
4. Roll your tacos; place them in preheated air fryer and cook at 350°F, for 6 minutes more. Divide fish tacos on plates and serve for breakfast

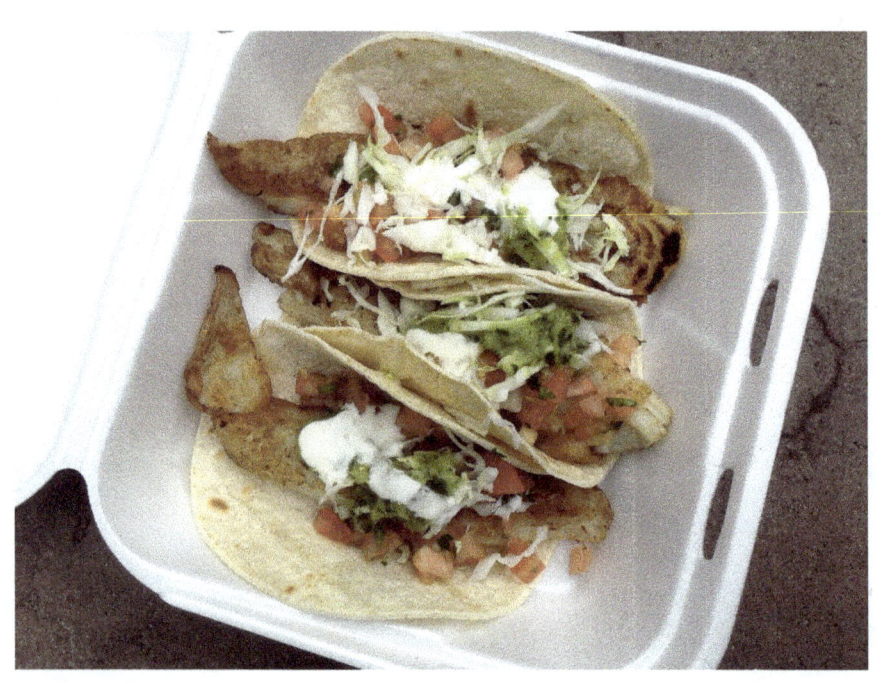

Tuna Sandwiches

Preparation Time: 14 minutes

Servings: 4

Ingredients:

- 16 oz. canned tuna; drained
- 6 bread slices
- 6 provolone cheese slices
- 2 spring onions; chopped.
- 1/4 cup mayonnaise
- 2 tbsp. mustard
- 1 tbsp. lime juice
- 3 tbsp. butter; melted

Directions:

1. In a bowl, mix the tuna, mayo, lime juice, mustard and spring onions; stir until combined.

2. Spread the bread slices with the butter, place them in preheated air fryer and bake them at 350°F for 5 minutes

3. Spread tuna mix on half of the bread slices and top with the cheese and the other bread slices
4. Place the sandwiches in your air fryer's basket and cook for 4 minutes more. Divide between plates and serve.

Tofu and Bell Peppers

Preparation Time: 15 minutes

Servings: 8

Ingredients:

- 3 oz. firm tofu; crumbled
- 1 green onion; chopped.
- 1 yellow bell pepper; cut into strips
- 1 orange bell pepper; cut into strips
- 1 green bell pepper; cut into strips
- 2 tbsp. parsley; chopped.
- Salt and black pepper to taste

Directions:

1. In a pan that fits your air fryer, place the bell pepper strips and mix
2. Then add all remaining ingredients, toss and place the pan in the air fryer. Cook at 400°F for 10 minutes. Divide between plates and serve

Cheering Chicken Sandwiches

Preparation Time: 20 Minutes

Servings: 4

Ingredients:

- 2 chicken breasts; skinless, boneless and cubed
- 1/2 cup Italian seasoning
- 1/2 tsp. thyme; dried
- 1 red onion; chopped.
- 1 red bell pepper; sliced
- 2 cups butter lettuce; torn
- 4 pita pockets
- 1 cup cherry tomatoes; halved
- 1 tbsp. olive oil

Directions:

1. In your air fryer, mix chicken with onion, bell pepper, Italian seasoning and oil; toss and cook at 380 °F, for 10 minutes.

Transfer chicken mix to a bowl; add thyme, butter lettuce and cherry tomatoes, toss well; stuff pita pockets with this mix and serve for lunch.

Nutrition Values: Calories: 126; Fat: 4; Fiber: 8; Carbs: 14; Protein: 4

Chicken Pie Recipe

Preparation Time: 29 Minutes

Servings: 4

Ingredients:

- 2 chicken thighs; boneless, skinless and cubed
- 1 carrot; chopped
- 1 tsp. Worcestershire sauce
- 1 tbsp. flour
- 1 tbsp. milk
- 2 puff pastry sheets
- 1 tbsp. butter; melted
- 1 yellow onion; chopped
- 2 potatoes; chopped
- 2 mushrooms; chopped
- 1 tsp. soy sauce
- Salt and black pepper to the taste
- 1 tsp. Italian seasoning
- 1/2 tsp. garlic powder

Directions:

1. Heat up a pan over medium high heat, add potatoes, carrots and onion; stir and cook for 2 minutes.
2. Add chicken and mushrooms, salt, soy sauce, pepper, Italian seasoning, garlic powder, Worcestershire sauce, flour and milk; stir really well and take off heat.
3. Place 1 puff pastry sheet on the bottom of your air fryer's pan and trim edge excess.
4. Add chicken mix, top with the other puff pastry sheet; trim excess as well and brush pie with butter.
5. Place in your air fryer and cook at 360 °F, for 6 minutes. Leave pie to cool down; slice and serve for breakfast.

Nutrition Values: Calories: 300; Fat: 5; Fiber: 7; Carbs: 14; Protein: 7

Dill and Scallops

Preparation Time: 15 Minutes

Servings: 4

Ingredients:

- 1 lb. sea scallops; debearded
- 1 tsp. dill; chopped.
- 2 tsp. olive oil
- 1 tbsp. lemon juice
- Salt and black pepper to the taste

Directions:

1. In your air fryer, mix scallops with dill, oil, salt, pepper and lemon juice; cover and cook at 360 °F, for 5 minutes. Discard unopened ones, divide scallops and dill sauce on plates and serve for lunch.

Nutrition Values: Calories: 152; Fat: 4; Fiber: 7; Carbs: 19; Protein: 4

Cheesy Ravioli and Marinara Sauce

Preparation Time: 18 Minutes

Servings: 6

Ingredients:

- 20 oz. cheese ravioli
- 10 oz. marinara sauce
- 1/4 cup parmesan; grated
- 1 tbsp. olive oil
- 1 cup buttermilk
- 2 cups bread crumbs

Directions:

1. Put buttermilk in a bowl and breadcrumbs in another bowl.

2. Dip ravioli in buttermilk, then in breadcrumbs and place them in your air fryer on a baking sheet. Drizzle olive oil over them; cook at 400 °F, for 5 minutes;

divide them on plates, sprinkle parmesan on top and serve for lunch

Nutrition Values: Calories: 270; Fat: 12; Fiber: 6; Carbs: 30; Protein: 15

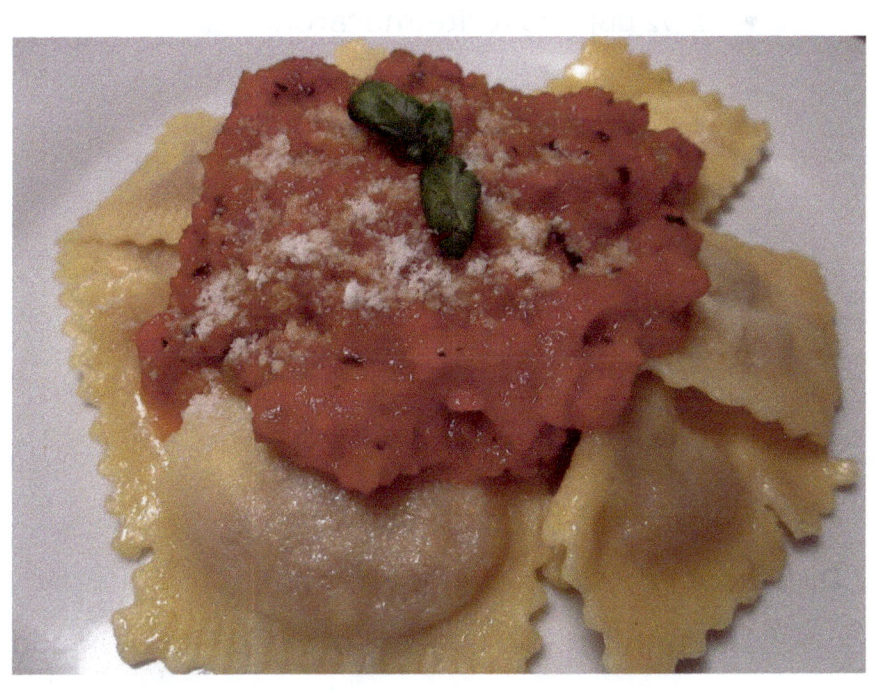

Cheese and Macaroni

Preparation Time: 40 Minutes

Servings: 3

Ingredients:

- 1 ½ cups favorite macaroni
- 1/2 cup heavy cream
- 1/2 cup mozzarella cheese; shredded
- 1/4 cup parmesan; shredded
- 1 cup chicken stock
- 3/4 cup cheddar cheese; shredded
- Salt and black pepper to the taste
- Cooking spray

Directions:

1. Spray a pan with cooking spray; add macaroni, heavy cream, stock, cheddar cheese, mozzarella and parmesan but also salt and pepper; toss well, place pan in your air fryer's basket and cook for 30 minutes. Divide among plates and serve for lunch.

Nutrition Values: Calories: 341; Fat: 7; Fiber: 8; Carbs: 18; Protein: 4

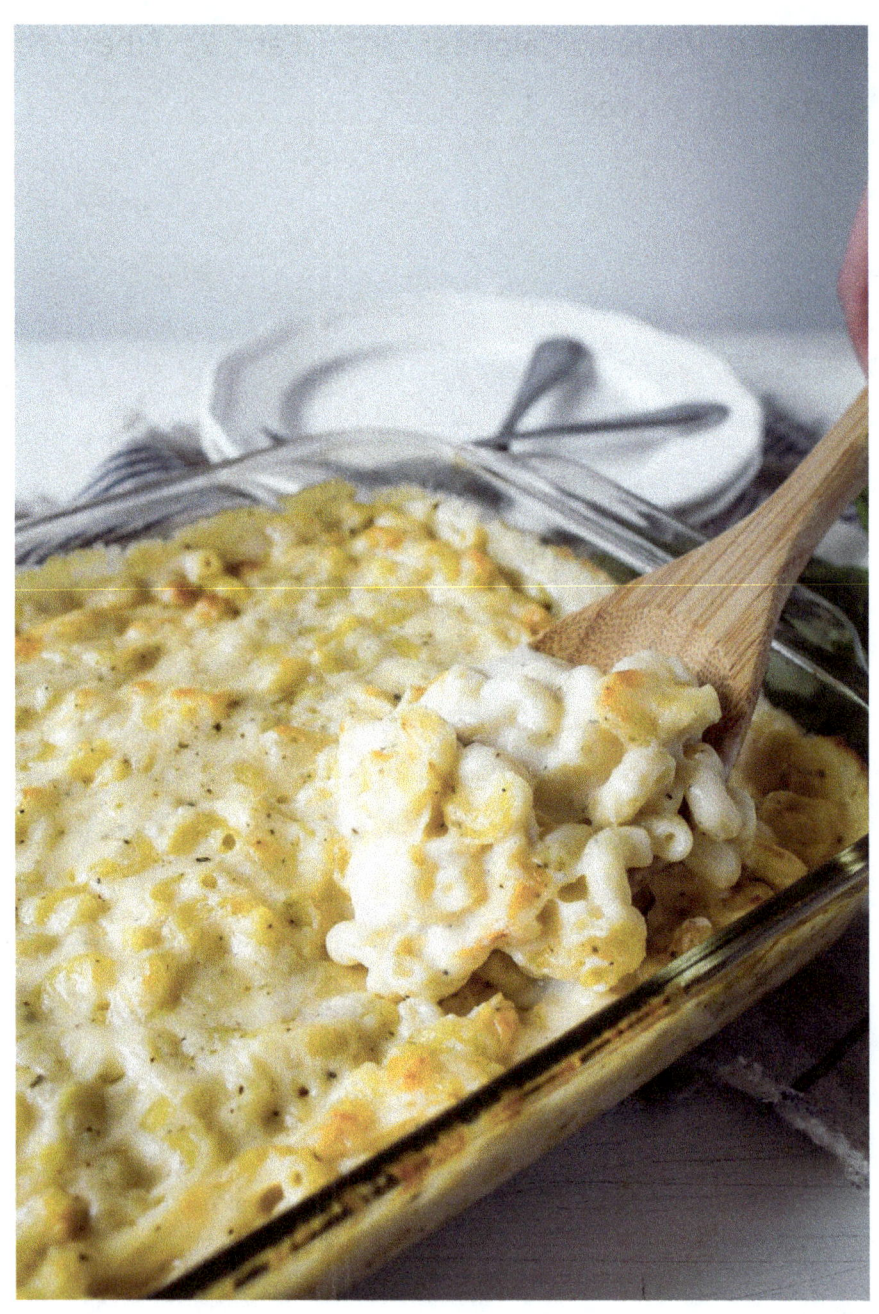

Zucchini and Tuna Tortillas

Preparation Time: 20 Minutes

Servings: 4

Ingredients:

- 1 cup zucchini; shredded
- 1/3 cup mayonnaise
- 2 tbsp. mustard
- 4 corn tortillas
- 4 tbsp. butter; soft
- 6 oz. canned tuna; drained
- 1 cup cheddar cheese; grated

Directions:

1. Spread butter on tortillas; place them in your air fryer's basket and cook them at 400 °F, for 3 minutes.
2. Meanwhile; in a bowl, mix tuna with zucchini, mayo and mustard and stir.

3. Divide this mix on each tortilla, top with cheese, roll tortillas; place them in your air fryer's basket again and cook them at 400 °F, for 4 minutes more. Serve for lunch.

Nutrition Values: Calories: 162; Fat: 4; Fiber: 8; Carbs: 9; Protein: 4

Beef Meatballs

Preparation Time: 25 Minutes

Servings: 4

Ingredients:

- 1/2 lb. beef; ground
- 1/2 tsp. garlic powder
- 1/2 tsp. onion powder
- 1/2 lb. Italian sausage; chopped.
- 1/2 cup cheddar cheese; grated
- Mashed potatoes for serving
- Salt and black pepper to the taste

Directions:

1. In a bowl; mix beef with sausage, garlic powder, onion powder, salt, pepper and cheese; stir well and shape 16 meatballs out of this mix.

2. Place meatballs in your air fryer and cook them at 370 °F, for 15 minutes. Serve your meatballs with some mashed potatoes on the side.

Nutrition Values: Calories: 333; Fat: 23; Fiber: 1; Carbs: 8; Protein: 20

Easy Egg Muffins

Preparation Time: 25 Minutes

Servings: 4

Ingredients:

- 2 tbsp. olive oil
- 3 tbsp. milk
- 1 egg
- 3.5 oz. white flour
- 1 tbsp. baking powder
- 2 oz. parmesan; grated
- A splash of Worcestershire sauce

Directions:

1. In a bowl; mix egg with flour, oil, baking powder, milk, Worcestershire and parmesan; whisk well and divide into 4 silicon muffin cups.

2. Arrange cups in your air fryer's cooking basket; cover and cook at 392, °F, for 15 minutes. Serve warm for breakfast.

Nutrition Values: Calories: 251; Fat: 6; Fiber: 8; Carbs: 9; Protein: 3

Breakfast Potatoes

Preparation Time: 45 Minutes

Servings: 4

Ingredients:

- 2 tbsp. olive oil
- 3 potatoes; cubed
- 1 yellow onion; chopped.
- 1 red bell pepper; chopped
- 1 tsp. garlic powder
- 1 tsp. sweet paprika
- 1 tsp. onion powder
- Salt and black pepper to the taste

Directions:

1. Grease your air fryer's basket with olive oil; add potatoes, toss and season with salt and pepper.

2. Add onion, bell pepper, garlic powder, paprika and onion powder, toss well, cover and cook at 370 °F, for 30 minutes. Divide potatoes mix on plates and serve for breakfast.

Nutrition Values: Calories: 214; Fat: 6; Fiber: 8; Carbs: 15; Protein: 4

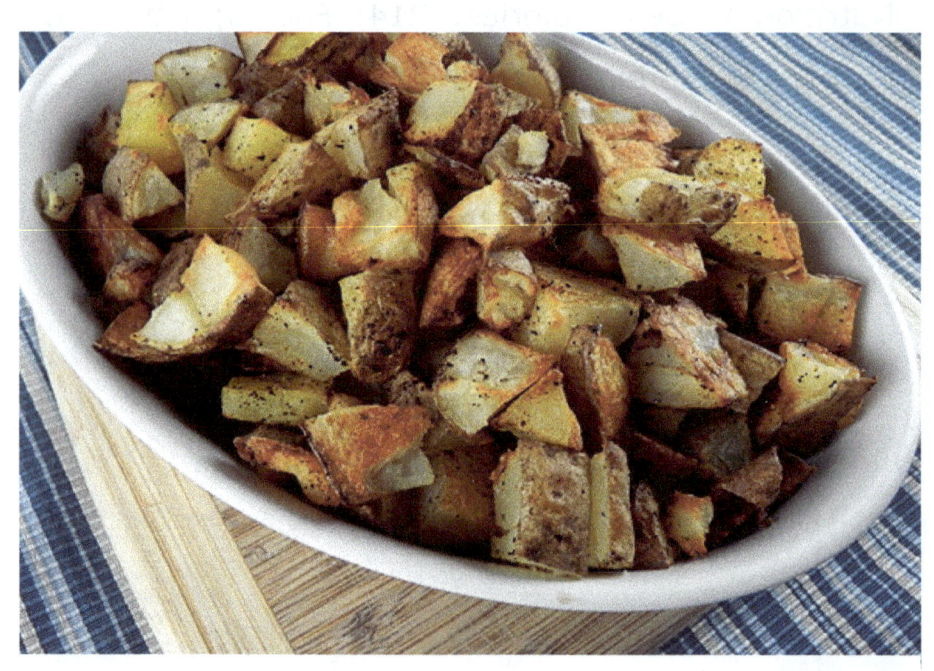

Breakfast Ham Dish

Preparation Time: 25 Minutes

Servings: 6

Ingredients:

- 6 cups French bread; cubed
- 4 oz. green chilies; chopped.
- 2 cups milk
- 5 eggs
- 1 tbsp. mustard
- 10 oz. ham; cubed
- 4 oz. cheddar cheese; shredded
- Salt and black pepper to the taste
- Cooking spray

Directions:

1. Heat up your air fryer at 350 °F and grease it with cooking spray.

2. In a bowl; mix eggs with milk, cheese, mustard, salt and pepper and stir.

3. Add bread cubes in your air fryer and mix with chilies and ham.
4. Add eggs mix; spread and cook for 15 minutes. Divide among plates and serve.

Nutrition Values: Calories: 200; Fat: 5; Fiber: 6; Carbs: 12; Protein: 14

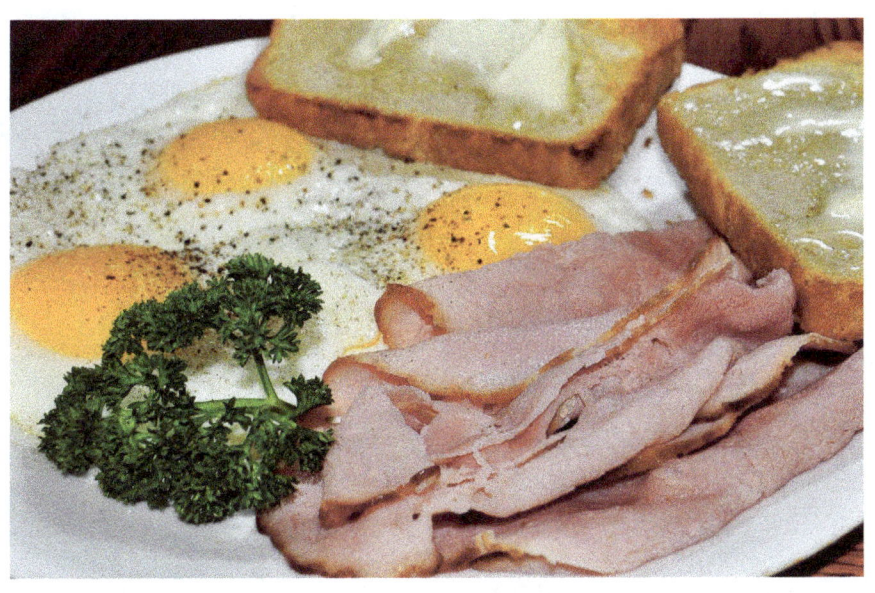

Banana Oatmeal Casserole

Preparation Time: 30 Minutes

Servings: 8

Ingredients:

- 2 cups rolled oats
- 1 tsp. baking powder
- 1/2 cup chocolate chips
- 2/3 cup blueberries
- 1 banana; peeled and mashed
- 1/3 cup brown sugar
- 1 tsp. cinnamon powder
- 2 cups milk
- 1 eggs
- 2 tbsp. butter
- 1 tsp. vanilla extract
- Cooking spray

Directions:

1. In a bowl; mix sugar with baking powder, cinnamon, chocolate chips, blueberries and banana and stir.
2. In a separate bowl; mix eggs with vanilla extract and butter and stir.
3. Heat up your air fryer at 320 degrees F; grease with cooking spray and add oats on the bottom.
4. Add cinnamon mix and eggs mix; toss and cook for 20 minutes. Stir one more time, divide into bowls and serve for breakfast.

Nutrition Values: Calories: 300; Fat: 4; Fiber: 7; Carbs: 12; Protein: 10

Tasty Polenta Bites

Preparation Time: 30 Minutes

Servings: 4

Ingredients:

For the polenta:

- 1 tbsp. butter
- 3 cups water
- 1 cup cornmeal
- Salt and black pepper to the taste

For the polenta bites:

- 2 tbsp. powdered sugar
- Cooking spray

Directions:

1. In a pan; mix water with cornmeal, butter, salt and pepper, stir, bring to a boil over medium heat; cook for 10 minutes, take off heat; whisk one more time and keep in the fridge until it's cold.

2. Scoop 1 tbsp. of polenta, shape a ball and place on a working surface.

3. Repeat with the rest of the polenta; arrange all the balls in the cooking basket of your air fryer, spray them with cooking spray; cover and cook at 380 °F, for 8 minutes. Arrange polenta bites on plates; sprinkle sugar all over and serve for breakfast.

Nutrition Values: Calories: 231; Fat: 7; Fiber: 8; Carbs: 12; Protein: 4

Eggs and Tomatoes

Preparation Time: 15 Minutes

Servings: 4

Ingredients:
- 4 eggs
- 2 oz. milk
- 2 tbsp. parmesan; grated
- 8 cherry tomatoes; halved
- Salt and black pepper to the taste
- Cooking spray

Directions:

1. Grease your air fryer with cooking spray and heat it up at 200 degrees F.
2. In a bowl; mix eggs with cheese, milk, salt and pepper and whisk.
3. Add this mix to your air fryer and cook for 6 minutes. Add tomatoes; cook your scrambled eggs for 3 minutes, divide among plates and serve.

Nutrition Values: Calories: 200; Fat: 4; Fiber: 7; Carbs: 12; Protein: 3

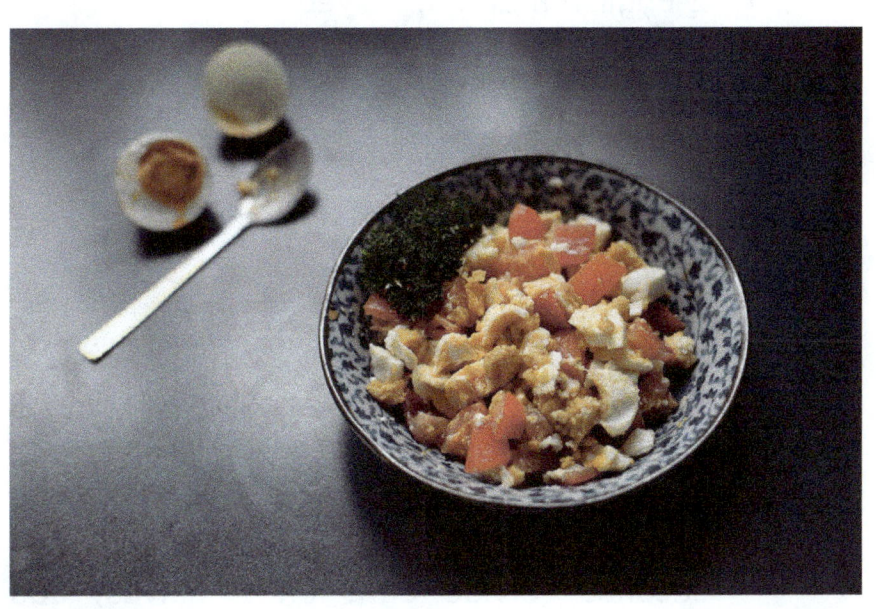

Fried Sandwich

Preparation Time: 16 Minutes

Servings: 2

Ingredients:

- 2 English muffins; halved
- 2 bacon strips
- 2 eggs
- Salt and black pepper to the taste

Preparation:

1. Crack eggs in your air fryer, add bacon on top; cover and cook at 392 °F, for 6 minutes. Heat up your English muffin halves in your microwave for a few seconds; divide eggs on 2 halves, add bacon on top, season with salt and pepper; cover with the other 2 English muffins and serve for breakfast.

Nutrition Values: Calories: 261; Fat: 5; Fiber: 8; Carbs: 12; Protein: 4

Breakfast Casserole

Preparation Time: 40 Minutes

Servings: 4

Ingredients:

- 3 tbsp. brown sugar
- 4 tbsp. butter
- 2 tbsp. white sugar
- 1/2 cup flour
- 1/2 tsp. cinnamon powder

For the casserole:

- 2 eggs
- 2 tbsp. white sugar
- 2 ½ cups white flour
- 1 tsp. baking soda
- 1 tsp. baking powder
- 2 eggs
- 1/2 cup milk
- 2 cups buttermilk

- 4 tbsp. butter
- 1 ⅔ cup blueberries
- Zest from 1 lemon; grated

Preparation:

1. In a bowl; mix eggs with 2 tbsp. white sugar, 2 ½ cups white flour, baking powder, baking soda, 2 eggs, milk, buttermilk, 4 tbsp. butter, lemon zest and blueberries; stir and pour into a pan that fits your air fryer.

2. In another bowls; mix 3 tbsp. brown sugar with 2 tbsp. white sugar, 4 tbsp. butter, 1/2 cup flour and cinnamon, stir until you obtain a crumble and spread over blueberries mix.

3. Place in preheated air fryer and bake at 300 °F, for 30 minutes. Divide among plates and serve for breakfast.

Nutrition Values: Calories: 214; Fat: 5; Fiber: 8; Carbs: 12; Protein: 5

Cheese Fried Bake

Preparation Time: 30 Minutes

Servings: 4

Ingredients:

- 4 bacon slices; cooked and crumbled
- 2 cups milk
- 1 lb. breakfast sausage; casings removed and chopped.
- 2 eggs
- 2 ½ cups cheddar cheese; shredded
- 1/2 tsp. onion powder
- 3 tbsp. parsley; chopped.
- Salt and black pepper to the taste
- Cooking spray

Directions:

1. In a bowl; mix eggs with milk, cheese, onion powder, salt, pepper and parsley and whisk well.

2. Grease your air fryer with cooking spray; heat it up at 320 °F and add bacon and sausage.
3. Add eggs mix; spread and cook for 20 minutes. Divide among plates and serve.

Nutrition Values: Calories: 214; Fat: 5; Fiber: 8; Carbs: 12; Protein: 12

Delightful Eggs Casserole

Preparation Time: 35 Minutes

Servings: 6

Ingredients:

- 12 eggs
- 1 lb. turkey; ground
- 1 sweet potato; cubed
- 1 cup baby spinach
- 1 tbsp. olive oil
- 1/2 tsp. chili powder
- 2 tomatoes; chopped for serving
- Salt and black pepper to the taste

Directions:

1. In a bowl; mix eggs with salt, pepper, chili powder, potato, spinach, turkey and sweet potato and whisk well.

2. Heat up your air fryer at 350 degrees F; add oil and heat it up.

3. Add eggs mix, spread into your air fryer; cover and cook for 25 minutes. Divide among plates and serve for breakfast.

Nutrition Values: Calories: 300; Fat: 5; Fiber: 8; Carbs: 13; Protein: 6

Morning Egg Bowls

Preparation Time: 30 Minutes

Servings: 4

Ingredients:

- 4 eggs
- 4 dinner rolls; tops cut off and insides scooped out
- 4 tbsp. mixed chives and parsley
- 4 tbsp. parmesan; grated
- 4 tbsp. heavy cream
- Salt and black pepper to the taste

Preparation:

1. Arrange dinner rolls on a baking sheet and crack an egg in each.
2. Divide heavy cream, mixed herbs in each roll and season with salt and pepper.
3. Sprinkle parmesan on top of your rolls; place them in your air fryer and cook at 350 °F, for 20 minutes. Divide your bread bowls on plates and serve for breakfast.

Nutrition Values: Calories: 238; Fat: 4; Fiber: 7; Carbs: 14; Protein: 7

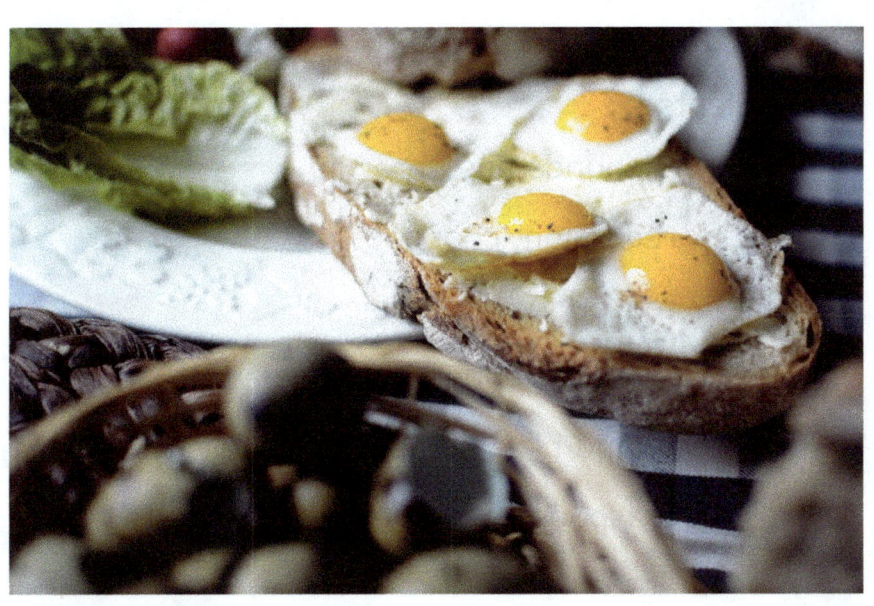

Thyme Potato Breakfast Mix

Preparation time: 5 minutes

Cooking time: 25 minutes

Servings: 4

Ingredients:

- 1½ pounds hash browns
- 1 red onion, chopped
- 2 teaspoons vegetable oil
- 1 red bell pepper, chopped
- Salt and black pepper to taste
- 1 teaspoon thyme, chopped
- 2 eggs

Directions:

1. Heat up your air fryer at 350 degrees F. Then add the oil and heat it up.

2. Add all other ingredients and cook for 25 minutes.

3. Divide between plates and serve

Nutrition Values: calories 241, fat 4, fiber 2, carbs 12, protein 11

Chicken and Spinach Breakfast Casserole

Preparation time: 5 minutes

Cooking time: 25 minutes

Servings: 4

Ingredients:

- 1 pound chicken meat, ground
- 1 tablespoon olive oil
- ½ teaspoon sweet paprika
- 12 eggs, whisked
- 1 cup baby spinach
- Salt and black pepper to taste

Directions:

1. In a bowl, whisk the eggs with the salt, pepper, and paprika. Then add the spinach and chicken and mix well.

2. Heat up your air fryer at 350 degrees F; add the oil and allow it to heat up.

3. Add the chicken and spinach mix, cover, and cook for 25 minutes.
4. Divide between plates and serve hot.

Nutrition Values: calories 270, fat 11, fiber 8, carbs 14, protein 7

Sausage Bake

Preparation time: 5 minutes

Cooking time: 20 minutes

Servings: 4

Ingredients:

- 4 bacon slices, cooked and crumbled
- A drizzle of olive oil
- 2 cups coconut milk
- 2½ cups cheddar cheese, shredded
- 1 pound breakfast sausage, chopped
- 2 eggs
- Salt and black pepper to taste
- 3 tablespoons cilantro, chopped

Directions:

1. In a bowl, mix the eggs with milk, cheese, salt, pepper, and the cilantro, and whisk well.

2. Grease your air fryer with the drizzle of oil, and heat it up at 320 degrees F.

3. Add the bacon, sausage, and the egg mixture, spread, and cook for 20 minutes.

4. Serve hot and enjoy!

Nutrition Values: calories 244, fat 11, fiber 8, carbs 15, protein 9

Breakfast Chicken Burrito

Preparation time: 5 minutes

Cooking time: 10 minutes

Servings: 2

Ingredients:

- 4 chicken breast slices, cooked and shredded
- 1 green bell pepper, sliced
- 2 eggs, whisked
- 1 avocado, peeled, pitted and sliced
- 2 tablespoons mild salsa
- Salt and black pepper to taste
- 2 tablespoons cheddar cheese, grated
- 2 tortillas

Directions:

1. In a bowl, whisk the eggs with the salt and pepper, and pour them into a pan that fits your air fryer.

2. Put the pan in the air fryer's basket, cook for 5 minutes at 400 degrees, and transfer the mix to a plate.
3. Place the tortillas on a working surface, and between them divide the eggs, chicken, bell peppers, avocado, and the cheese; roll the burritos.
4. Line your air fryer with tin foil, add the burritos, and cook them at 300 degrees F for 3-4 minutes.
5. Serve for breakfast—or lunch, or dinner!

Nutrition Values: calories 329, fat 13, fiber 11, carbs 20, protein 8

Fruity Breakfast Casserole

Preparation time: 10 minutes

Cooking time: 20 minutes

Servings: 6

Ingredients:

- 2 cups old fashioned oats
- 1 teaspoon baking powder
- ⅓ cup sugar
- 1 teaspoon cinnamon powder
- 1 cup blueberries
- 1 banana, peeled and mashed
- 2 cups milk
- 2 eggs, whisked
- 2 tablespoons butter
- 1 teaspoon vanilla extract
- Cooking spray

Directions:

1. In a bowl, mix the sugar, baking powder, cinnamon, blueberries, banana, eggs, butter, and vanilla; whisk.

2. Heat up your air fryer at 320 degrees F, and grease with cooking spray.

3. Add the oats, the berries and banana mix; cover, and cook for 20 minutes.

4. Divide into bowls and serve.

Nutrition Values: calories 260, fat 4, fiber 7, carbs 9, protein 10

Smoked Bacon and Bread Mix

Preparation time: 10 minutes

Cooking time: 30 minutes

Servings: 6

Ingredients:

- 1 pound white bread, cubed
- 1 pound smoked bacon, cooked and chopped
- ¼ cup avocado oil
- 1 red onion, chopped
- 30 ounces canned tomatoes, chopped
- ½ pound cheddar cheese, shredded
- 2 tablespoons chives, chopped
- ½ pound Monterey jack cheese, shredded
- 2 tablespoons chicken stock
- Salt and black pepper to taste
- 8 eggs, whisked

Directions:

1. Add the oil to your air fryer and heat it up at 350 degrees F.

2. Add all other ingredients except the chives and cook for 30 minutes, shaking halfway.

3. Divide between plates and serve with chives sprinkled on top.

Nutrition Values: calories 211, fat 8, fiber 7, carbs 14, protein 3

Cheesy Hash Brown Mix

Preparation time: 10 minutes

Cooking time: 20 minutes

Servings: 6

Ingredients:

- 1½ pounds hash browns
- 1 cup almond milk
- A drizzle of olive oil
- 6 bacon slices, chopped
- 8 ounces cream cheese, softened
- 1 yellow onion, chopped
- 1 cup cheddar cheese, shredded
- 6 spring onions, chopped
- Salt and black pepper to taste
- 6 eggs

Directions:

1. Heat up your air fryer with the oil at 350 degrees F.

2. In a bowl, mix all other ingredients except the spring onions, and whisk well.
3. Add this mixture to your air fryer, cover, and cook for 20 minutes.
4. Divide between plates, sprinkle the spring onions on top, and serve.

Nutrition Values: calories 231, fat 9, fiber 9, carbs 8, protein 12

Roasted Peppers Frittata

Preparation time: 10 minutes

Cooking time: 20 minutes

Servings: 6

Ingredients:

- 6 ounces jarred roasted red bell peppers, chopped
- 12 eggs, whisked
- ½ cup parmesan cheese, grated
- 3 garlic cloves, minced
- 2 tablespoons parsley, chopped
- Salt and black pepper to taste
- 2 tablespoons chives, chopped
- 6 tablespoons ricotta cheese
- A drizzle of olive oil

Directions:

1. In a bowl, mix the bell peppers with the eggs, garlic, parsley, salt, pepper, chives, and ricotta; whisk well.

2. Heat up your air fryer at 300 degrees F, add the oil, and spread.
3. Add the egg mixture, spread, sprinkle the parmesan on top, and cook for 20 minutes.
4. Divide between plates and serve.

Nutrition Values: calories 262, fat 6, fiber 9, carbs 18, protein 8

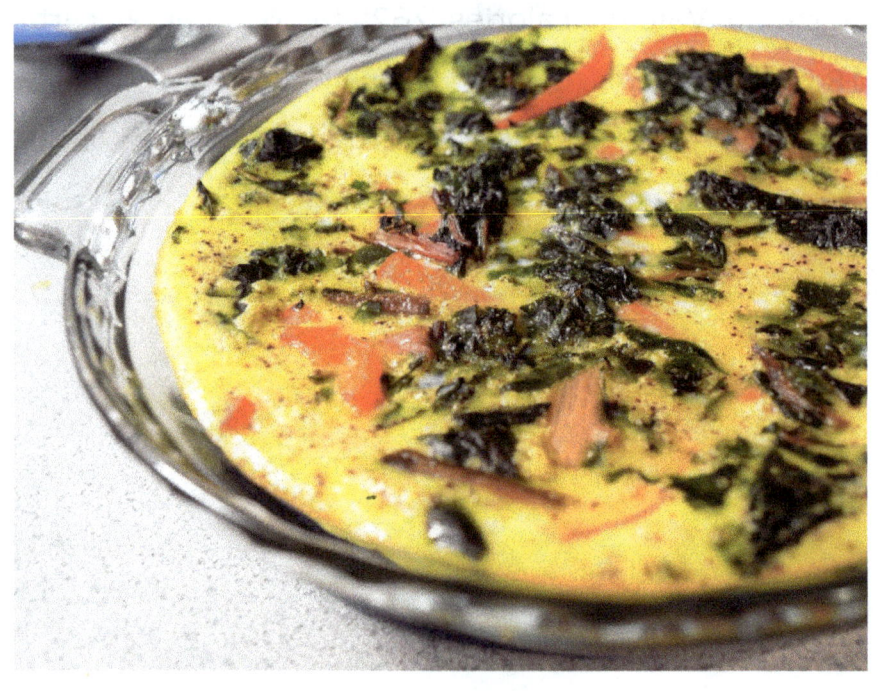

Blackberries and Cornflakes Mix

Preparation time: 5 minutes

Cooking time: 10 minutes

Servings: 4

Ingredients:

- 3 cups milk
- 1 tablespoon sugar
- 2 eggs, whisked
- ¼ teaspoon nutmeg, ground
- ¼ cup blackberries
- 4 tablespoons cream cheese, whipped
- 1½ cups corn flakes

Directions:

1. In a bowl, mix all ingredients and stir well.
2. Heat up your air fryer at 350 degrees F, add the corn flakes mixture, spread, and cook for 10 minutes.

3. Divide between plates, serve, and enjoy.

Nutrition Values: calories 180, fat 5, fiber 7, carbs 12, protein 5

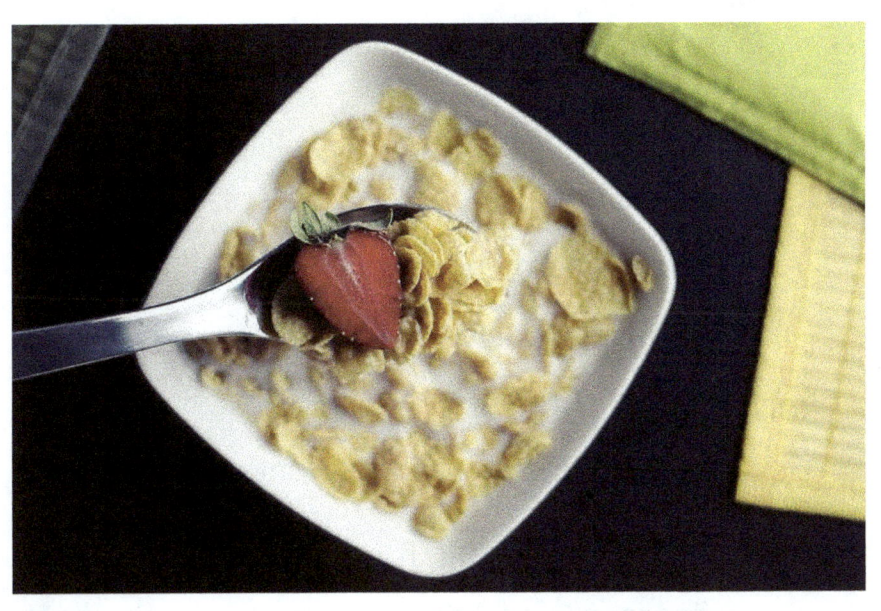

Simple Scrambled Eggs

Preparation time: 5 minutes

Cooking time: 10 minutes

Servings: 4

Ingredients:

- 4 eggs, whisked
- A drizzle of olive oil
- Salt and black pepper to taste
- 1 red onion, chopped
- 2 teaspoons sweet paprika

Directions:

1. In a bowl, mix all ingredients and whisk.
2. Heat up your air fryer with the oil at 240 degrees F, add the eggs mixture, stir again, and cook for 10 minutes.
3. Serve right away.

Nutrition Values: calories 190, fat 7, fiber 7, carbs 12, protein 4

Creamy Mushroom Pie

Preparation time: 10 minutes

Cooking time: 10 minutes

Servings: 4

Ingredients:

- 1 tablespoon olive oil
- 9-inch pie dough
- 6 white mushrooms, chopped
- 2 tablespoons bacon, cooked and crumbled
- 3 eggs
- 1 red onion, chopped
- ½ cup heavy cream
- Salt and black pepper to taste
- ½ teaspoon thyme, dried
- ¼ cup cheddar cheese, grated

Directions:

1. Roll the dough on a working surface, then press it on the bottom of a pie pan that fits your air fryer and grease with the oil.

2. In a bowl, mix all other ingredients except the cheese, stir well, and pour mixture into the pie pan.
3. Sprinkle the cheese on top, put the pan in the air fryer, and cook at 400 degrees F for 10 minutes.
4. Slice and serve.

Nutrition Values: calories 192, fat 6, fiber 6, carbs 14, protein 7

Carrots and Cauliflower Breakfast Mix

Preparation time: 10 minutes

Cooking time: 20 minutes

Servings: 4

Ingredients:

- 1 cauliflower head, stems removed, florets separated, and steamed
- 3 carrots, chopped and steamed
- 2 ounces cheddar cheese, grated
- 3 eggs
- 2 ounces milk
- 2 teaspoons cilantro, chopped
- Salt and black pepper to taste

Directions:

1. In a bowl, mix the eggs with the milk, parsley, salt, and pepper; whisk.

2. Put the cauliflower and the carrots in your air fryer, add the egg mixture, and spread. Then sprinkle the cheese on top.
3. Cook at 350 degrees F for 20 minutes, divide between plates, and serve.

Nutrition Values: calories 194, fat 4, fiber 7, carbs 11, protein 6

Delicious Doughnuts

Preparation Time: 28 Minutes

Servings: 6

Ingredients:

- 1/2 cup sugar
- 2 ¼ cups white flour
- 1 tsp. cinnamon powder
- 2 egg yolks
- 1/3 cup caster sugar
- 4 tbsp. butter; soft
- 1 ½ tsp. baking powder
- 1/2 cup sour cream

Directions:

1. In a bowl; mix 2 tablespoon butter with simple sugar and egg yolks and whisk well
2. Add half of the sour cream and stir.
3. In another bowls; mix flour with baking powder, stir and also add to eggs mix

4. Stir well until you obtain a dough, transfer it to a floured working surface; roll it out and cut big circles with smaller ones in the middle.

5. Brush doughnuts with the rest of the butter; heat up your air fryer at 360 degrees F; place doughnuts inside and cook them for 8 minutes

6. In a bowl; mix cinnamon with caster sugar and stir. Arrange doughnuts on plates and dip them in cinnamon and sugar before serving.

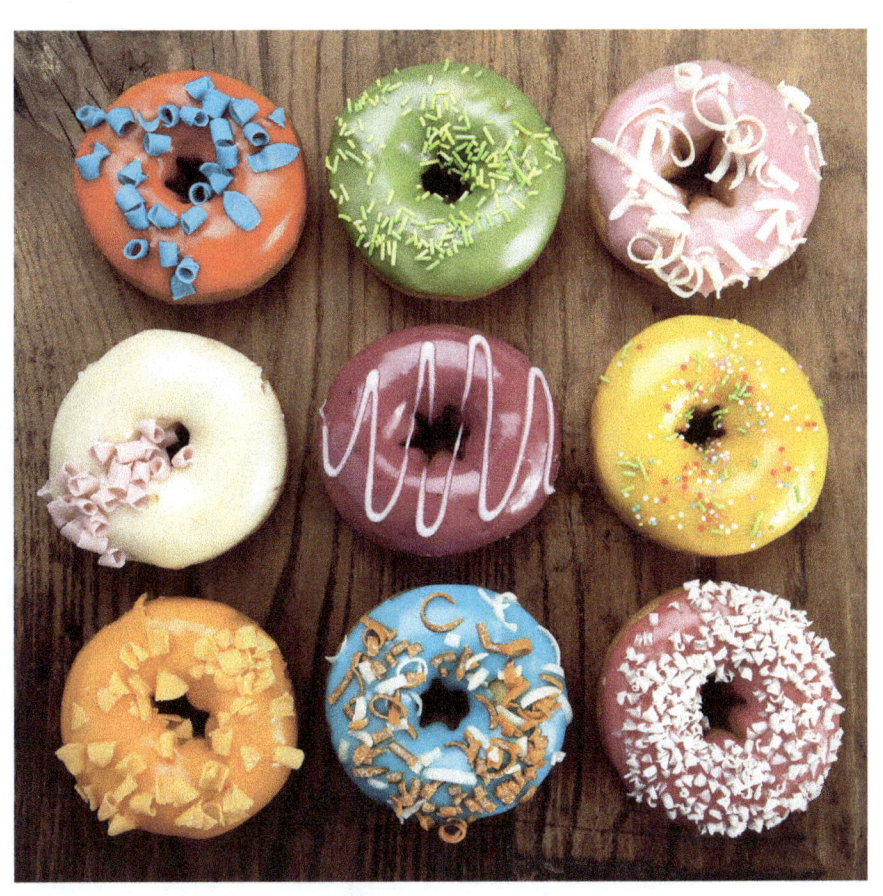

www.ingramcontent.com/pod-product-compliance
Lightning Source LLC
Chambersburg PA
CBHW070730030426
42336CB00013B/1934